Whole Foods Diet Phenomenon

Plant Based Diet 101

By Cathy Wilson
Copyright © 2013

Income Disclaimer

This book contains business strategies, marketing methods and other business advice that, regardless of my own results and experience, may not produce the same results (or any results) for you. I make absolutely no guarantee, expressed or implied, that by following the advice below you will make any money or improve current profits, as there are several factors and variables that come into play regarding any given business.

Primarily, results will depend on the nature of the product or business model, the conditions of the marketplace, the experience of the individual, and situations and elements that are beyond your control.

As with any business endeavor, you assume all risk related to investment and money based on your own discretion and at your own potential expense.

Liability Disclaimer

By reading this book, you assume all risks associated with using the advice given below, with a full understanding that you, solely, are responsible for anything that may occur as a result of putting this information into action in any way, and regardless of your interpretation of the advice.

You further agree that our company cannot be held responsible in any way for the success or failure of your business as a result of the information presented in this book. It is your responsibility to conduct your own due diligence regarding the safe and successful operation of your business if you intend to apply any of our information in any way to your business operations.

Terms of Use

You are given a non-transferable, "personal use" license to this book. You cannot distribute it or share it with other individuals.

Also, there are no resale rights or private label rights granted when purchasing this book. In other words, it's for your own personal use only.

Whole Foods Diet Phenomenon

Plant Based Diet 101

By Cathy Wilson

Table of Contents

Introduction

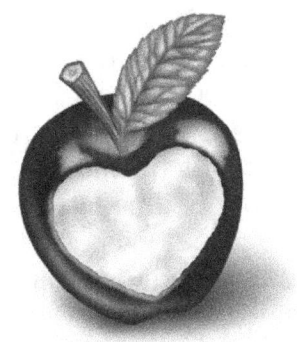

Whole Foods Plant Based Diet eating will . . .

* Enable more efficient BRAIN function
* Help deter the deterioration of your Body and build it strong
* Encourage a healthy and stable WEIGHT
* Ease your MIND and reduce STRESS just knowing you are eating natural
* Remind your TASTEBUDS that healthy eating is REAL flavor

Are you going to keep allowing extrinsic societal pressures to determine your destiny? Are you going to take control of your own well-being and make the decision to get back with nature and implement healthy and wholesome Whole Foods Plant Based eating into your everyday?

We live in a crazy fast paced world that leaves little room for au natural. The faster the better and this means modified foods too. People aren't conditioned these days to make time to prepare natural and wholesome foods to eat because it's so much easier to scoot through the drive thru on your way to work and grab an unhealthy egg sandwich. Instead of making the time to grab some fresh fruit from a garden market, we just pop a few coins into the vending machine and down a pastry instead. A decision like that here or there really isn't going to cause an issue. What happens is that we are lazy and these actions quickly manifest into habit. Over time, this decision will interfere with your good health and the ability for your mind and body to function optimally, to carry you through life lean and fit, healthy and energetic, and strong until the end of the line.

Poor eating habits and little or no regular exercise. results in obesity, which triggers all sorts of serious health issues including diabetes, stroke and cardiovascular disease to start. These are health issues that steal your quality of life and more and for the most part are absolute. The sad part is this is mostly preventable and if we, as a society could wake up and smell the pure water instead of the coffee, life would bring a whole lot more smiles all around.

Choosing to get healthy by going back in time to exercising regularly and making Whole Food Plant Based Diet choices for eating, is going to turn your world right-side-up.

You will:
* Lose fat for good
* Gain energy
* Become more productive
* Decrease mood swings
* Think with clarity
* Lower the risk of serious disease
* Give you that "feel good" feeling we all crave

* Ease stress just knowing you are eating healthy
The bottom line is that by implementing Whole Foods Plant Based Diet into your everyday along with a healthy exercise regimen you WILL succeed in long-term weight loss and overall great health and wellness. Are you ready to get started?

Whole Foods Explained

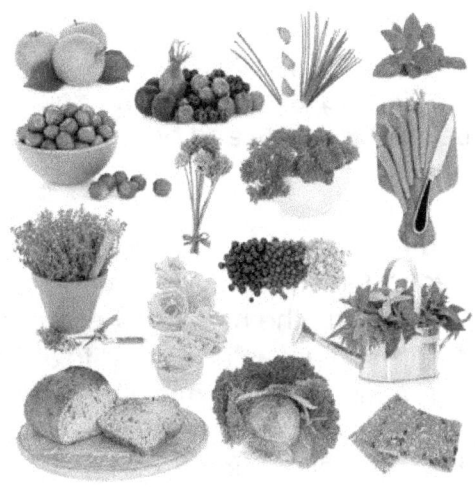

Whole foods are foods which are all natural, unprocessed and unrefined as much as possible. Avoid additives and preservatives, including added fat, salt and carbohydrates. Rewinding time, all foods used to be whole, including unpasteurized milk products. Experts agree that food processing which involves the addition of numerous chemicals and preservatives, negatively impacts your health. Heart disease, high blood pressure, cancer, stroke and many other serious diseases are linked to foods that have been chemically altered through processing.

Rule of Thumb - If the food isn't packaged and doesn't come with an ingredient list, it's in a natural state with nothing added, then chances are pretty good you're making a healthy choice.

Some are confused that whole foods are always organic. *Organic foods are produced, manufactured and handled following the USDA guide with regards to organic foods. Natural or Whole foods are not mandated by this process.*

The bottom line is an organic food isn't always whole and a whole food isn't always organic. Am I confusing you? Just remember whole foods and organic foods should be your first choice!

Enzymes found in whole foods are critical in all chemical processes in your body, particularly when it comes to digesting food. If you add the heating of processed foods, chemicals and preservatives and other toxins to the mix, then you are creating more chemical reactions which are volatile and destructive, taking away the health benefits of the foods you are consuming.

These triggered unnatural chemical reactions have dangerous effects on your health,even just cooking some foods can create negative chemical reactions. For instance, heating carbohydrates like in processed and packaged high-fat simple carbs can transform into carcinogens called acrylamide, which is a chemical used in plastics and dyes and causes cancer in animals.

Today we want convenience and have conditioned ourselves to ignore healthy whole foods and opt for the sugar laden, high-fat, unhealthy "fast" foods, all of which interfere with the smooth running of your intricate bodily systems, creating disease, illness and eventually death.

This isn't something you can fix with a band-aid. If you want to gain control of your health, it's time to make the commitment to do it right. This means you've got to make the mental, physical and emotional changes to make whole food eating your new "normal."

Is this going to take time? That's a big YES. Are you going to need patience, perseverance, support and expert knowledge to do it? That's affirmative. By understanding what whole foods are and how they can benefit your health, mind, body and soul, you will see that making the switch to whole food eating really is a no-brainer.

Don't try and be perfect here. Change is hard. Take it one step at a time and set yourself up for success. Learn to implement manageable changes that will stick for your lifetime. Seeing is believing for most of us and slowly, but surely, you will look and feel differently and this will fuel your desire to make more positive changes in your eating. That's just the way the cookie crumbles, or should I say banana gets peeled?

Whole foods used to be the only way people ate because there was no choice. Now we have choice and it's up to you to make your own decision. You can continue eating processed and unhealthy toxic foods that are "knowingly" destroying your body and mind from the inside out, or you can choose to step up to the plate to make a positive lifestyle change. Start making whole food choices and begin experiencing what healthy eating is all about. How does that sound to you?

When you are pondering different whole foods just think about foods that are closest to their natural state. A baked potato is a whole food, French fries are NOT! Just to be certain, here's a list of some whole foods you may or may not have thought about.

Examples Whole Foods
* Fresh fruits and vegetables

* Fresh herbs
* Grains - wheat, oats, rice, barley, corn and spelt
* Unpasteurized milk and milk products
* Free-Range meats void of chemicals, preservatives, hormones and medicines

NOTE: The further grains go along in the refining process the less likely they're going to classified as a "whole" food. The more processed they are the less nutrition they have.

My Thoughts . . .
Understanding what whole foods are, is important in establishing a solid base from which to build and implement our healthy eating strategy. There is a difference between organic and whole foods, but both are your best route to good health, less disease and greater energy. The choice is yours.

Benefits of Eating Whole Foods

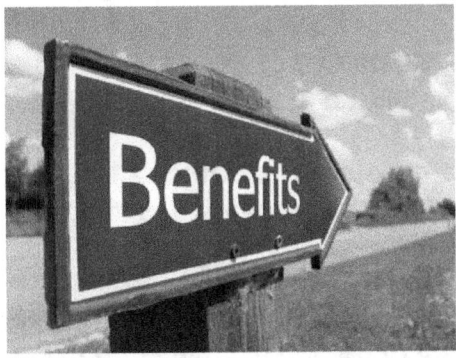

The more we dig past the surface of nutrition and healthy eating, the more sense it makes to eat the way our ancestors did hundreds of years ago, fueling their bodies with all natural wholesome foods straight from nature, void of harmful processing, chemicals and preservatives that are scientifically proven to interfere with good health mentally and physically.

It's not always practical to eat whole foods, but the idea is not to be perfect here, rather to aim to consume whole foods as much as you can. This is beneficial to your body and mind in so many different ways. Eating whole foods means . . .

* Choosing whole grains instead of processed and refined - *brown instead of white*

* Filling your plate full of fresh fruits, vegetables and wholesome beans instead of depending on supplementation - *the real deal instead of pill popping*

* Smoothie drinks made with fresh fruits and vegetables rather than store juice or sugared slush drinks - *natural instead of processed sugars*

* Grilled free-range chicken instead of deep fried chicken nuggets - *natural meats void of hormones and other chemicals instead of high fat chicken with less nutrients and lots of additives*

* Baked sweet potato instead of a bag of potato chips *- all natural complex carbohydrates instead of nutritionless processed simple carbohydrates*

* Dish of fresh fruit unsweetened instead of a fruit pastry - *Loads of natural vitamins and minerals instead of processed high fat, calorie loaded and no nutrient sweets*

* Green tea instead of soda - natural *beverage with numerous health benefits instead of a big glass of sugar that gives you a hyper high which sets you up for a depressing fall*

* Apple or pear instead of a fruit snack - whole and healthy simple carbohydrate with energy and nutrient rich sugars, instead of processed fruit snacks with lots of sugars, additives and little nutritional value.

Experts agree that eating more natural whole foods is your direct route to better health, more energy, less fat and avoiding or at least deterring disease. Choose fresh fruits and vegetables, whole grains, legumes and nuts are whole foods that have plenty of fiber and nutrients that are often lost in processing. Hugely beneficial phytochemicals are often lost during the processing process.

Whole food eating is beginning to make a comeback and this is music to health expert's ears and yours too! Let's have a gander at a few reasons whole foods should be making their way to your belly:

Nutrient Advantage

Experts report that a large portion of the population gets too little Vitamin C and A, potassium, fiber and magnesium to start. The fact is that disease studies show people who get adequate amounts of these vitamins and minerals in specific, lower their risk considerably of developing heart disease, high blood pressure and cholesterol, diabetes and cancer. Of course whole food eating tops up your stores and ensures you are level on the nutrient playing field.

The majority of missing nutrients in your diet can simply be rectified with a whole food - plant based eating strategy. It's not just me yapping away here because nutritionists agree.

Essential Phytochemicals

What are Phytochemicals? They are simply chemical substances naturally found in plants that aim to prevent free radicals from manifesting within your body and producing disease through cell damage. Scientists are discovering new phytochemicals regularly and right now there are in excess of 1,000 known.

If you want phytochemicals you need to eat plant-based foods in their natural state. Processing them often zaps their disease-preventing benefits. Lycopene is found in red colored phytochemical found in foods like tomatoes and red peppers. Anthocyanins give the marvelous blue color to berries and pterostilbene is a powerful antioxidant that seems to trigger the cells in berries and grapes to metabolize fat and cholesterol.

In order to take advantage of these protective chemicals you need to fill your body full of whole foods.

Healthy Fats

Trans fats and saturated fats are what we need to steer clear of when healthy eating is our focus. Processed and packaged foods are loaded with these "bad" fats, making it very difficult to lose weight and even easier to develop disease. Whole foods have very little if any "bad" fat.

They have healthy fats in moderate amounts and this is exactly what your body requires to find that perfect balance of maintaining energy and metabolizing nasty fat. Good fats also help with deterring disease and improving brain function. Unsaturated fats like sunflower oil, avocado and olive oil should be your fats of choice for optimal health.

Wholesome Fiber

Wholesome fiber is abundant in most whole foods, where it's lost in the processing of most foods. Fiber really helps benefit your healthy by:

* Making you feel full faster
* Lower the risk of diabetes and heart disease
* Moves your GI tract along
Fiber-rich foods help control blood sugars, fat and weight, according to health and wellness experts. Ridding your body of harmful toxins is a necessity of good health and eating whole foods is a great start.

Whole Grains

Whole grain foods not only have loads of fiber, but they also have so many nutrients vital to great health. Switching to whole grain foods lowers your risk of developing diabetes and lower cholesterol and blood pressure. Adipose tissue - the fat tissue around your organs and muscles - is shown in lower levels when people chose whole grains over refined.

Less "Extras"

Whole foods do not have preservatives, chemicals or harmful hormones added. The "extras" that allow processed foods to last so long on the shelf and taste so sweet. These "extras" make foods somewhat addictive and easy to make habit. Eat whole foods, and you'll eliminate the harmful "extras" that directly trigger disease and interfere with good health.

Other Benefits of Whole Foods

Reduces the risk of cataracts, which is a clouding over of the lens of the eye found in over half of people over 75
Reduces the amino acid homocysteine , which is often accumulated to high levels in people that don't eat healthy, increasing the risk of cardiovascular disease and stroke
Healthy isoflavones and lignans are phytonutrients found in whole foods like berries and flaxseed that studies suggest lower the risk for cancers of the reproductive system.

TAKE ACTION! Tips for Incorporating Whole Foods Into Your Life

* When it comes to whole grains, breads and starches make sure you choose 100% whole grains without preservatives. Natural whole grains will spoil faster than with

additives. If bread can last up to two weeks, then it has something added. However, if a whole grain bread expires in a few days, chances are pretty good that it's full of whole grain goodness. Be sure to read the label to be sure.

* If your tummy is grumbling for a snack go for fresh fruits and vegetables. Always have them prepped and ready in the fridge so when you're hungry you don't have to worry about cutting them up. Often, that's just enough of a deterrent to set your sites on the snack cupboard. Filling your plate at mealtime with plenty of sweet and tasty vegetables is also important. This is going to fill you up because of the fiber, protect you from disease because of the antioxidants, help burn fat and give you ample energy to make it that will build up and manifest into disease over time.

* If you are a baker you can start substituting whole grain flour for traditional white. Start with half and half because some recipes don't do so well with all whole grain. Better yet, start switching to tasty all-natural whole grain recipes. Often they are tastier anyway. Change is good!

* Scale back on the high fat, little nutrients, calorie loaded processed and packaged convenience foods. All these are going to do is fill your body and blood full, and blood full of harmful fats that are going to slow your systems down, stress your body with extra fat stores, zap your confidence and leave you uninspired for life.

* Try and eat more beans as snacks and with meals. They are full of fiber, plant protein, heart healthy phytochemicals and numerous other essential nutrients. Beans help build lean muscle and fuel your body for long term energy that lasts. Beans are flavorful, inexpensive and versatile.

Adzuki Beans are little sweet red beans that are easy on the digestive system and taste fabulous with brown rice and celery for excellent protein and fiber rich patties. Chick peas are used often in the Mediterranean and are great for taming potent spices, adding to chili, soups and salads.

Kidney Beans are very popular in chili, casseroles, soups, salads and stir fry's. Just be sure to fully cook them, otherwise they are nasty hard.

Those are just a few examples of how you can use tasty, nutrient and fiber dense beans to your advantage.

Did You Know?
Tongues of Fire and Mortgage Lifters are a few of the crazy named beans available throughout the United States!

My Thoughts . . .
It's fair to say the benefit of whole food plant based eating is endless. Technically we should shoot for 100% percent whole food eating, but that's just not practical. We all lead hectic lives full of daily stresses and with limited time comes the need for convenience. Unfortunately, grabbing unhealthy processed fast foods seems to be the norm, turning into habit quickly and this ends up being one un-healthy energy stealing, fat fueling, disease triggering habit to break. Science says whole foods are best. Medical professionals agree. Good luck finding any health and wellness expert that isn't on board with wholesome and healthy whole food eating. Need I say more?

What Nutrients Do Plants Provide?

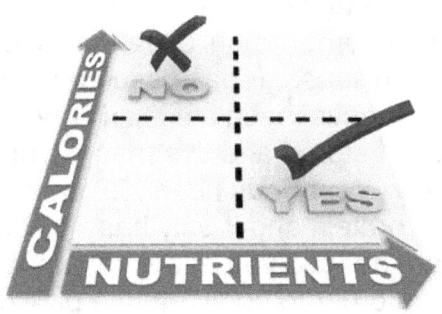

In order to be healthy and happy and have a body that functions optimally and a mind that's sharp and clear, you need certain nutrients. The six basic nutrients your body needs are:

* Carbohydrates
* Protein
* Fat
* Vitamins
* Minerals
* Water

Carbohydrates are required for energy, breaking down protein, and for protecting your body from harmful toxins. Complex carbohydrates are what you need because the glucose in them is critical to good health. Whole grains and vegetables are great sources, with starch as an important component in the big picture of good health. *Servings - 6-8/day*

Avoiding high sugar, high fat, simple refined sugar carbohydrates with very little nutrients is important.

Sources: White bread, white pasta and rice, pastries,
cookies, chocolate bars and candy

Protein is an important macronutrient your body needs in
large quantities in order to build lean muscle, regulate
hormones, fight disease, repair tissue and provide energy. Protein is essential because it isn't manufactured by
the body, nor is it stored and this means you need to
consume it daily. Your body needs 22 amino acids in order to produce protein and it only has 14 naturally. This
means through the food you eat, eight amino acids must
be consumed in order to complete the protein your body
needs to thrive.

Sources: Various meats, fish, chicken, dairy products,
eggs, nuts, beans and quinoa

**Note: When choosing lean meats for whole food eat-
ing you should look for meats that are void of
hormones, antibiotics or other drugs and fed an organic diet that steers clear of pesticides and other
harmful toxins. Au natural is what you're looking for.**

Servings - 2-3/day

Fat is something you simply can't live without. The two
basic types are saturated and unsaturated. Fat provides
more energy that both macronutrients protein and carbohydrates, helps with vitamin absorption, keeps you warm,
levels temperature and protects your vital organs. Saturated fats like butter and lard interfere with your good
health and contribute to obesity and serious disease
when consumed in large amounts. Trans fat is even more
dangerous than saturated because it's chemically altered

so food has more flavor, stability and a longer shelf life to start. Processed foods often have these BAD fats.

Sources of GOOD fats: Avocado, olive oil, sunflower oil and olive oil

Servings - Most of us don't need to worry about getting enough fat in our diet, but focus on eating good fats not bad ones, along with cutting back. Less than 30% of your daily caloric intake should come from fats. No more than 10% should come from saturated fats.

Vitamins are essentially chemicals your body requires to process vital nutrients, build genes, red bloods cells, proteins and hormones and to regulate your central nervous system. By eating a diverse diet filled with plenty of fresh fruits and vegetables, lean meats, low fat dairy products and complex carbohydrates you should be able to provide your body with adequate amounts of vitamins to maintain optimal health.

Sources: Poultry, fish, dairy, lean meat, eggs, fruits and vegetables

Minerals are important in keeping your body and mind strong. These are inorganic substances your body requires for making bones, teeth, body fluid regulation, generating blood cells and assisting in natural chemical processes. There are two main types of essential minerals; Macronutrients and micronutrients.

Macro includes protein, carbohydrates and fat.
Micro, which the body needs in small amounts, includes zinc, copper, cobalt, iron, iodine, manganese, fluoride, molybdenum and selenium.

Eating a healthy well balanced diet should provide adequate amounts of micronutrients.

Water is hands down the most important component for your body. Up to 75% of your body is water. So it makes sense 6-8 glasses of day of pure, natural and tasty water is required to help your internal bodily systems run smoothly. Water helps to purge toxins from your body, maintain skin, nails and hair, help with digestion and transport vital nutrients throughout your body via the bloodstream. Water hydrates you and gives you energy to function throughout the day. If you don't get enough water you will become dehydrating, leaving you feeling fatigued, lethargic and in extreme cases this can even cause confused thinking.

Of course, if you are exercising regularly you need to drink more because your body is burning more energy. Keep in mind there is a difference between a soda and glass of water. Your best choices are water, herbal teas and clear soups. Sodas are just full of excess sugars directly linked to obesity and disease.

Servings - 6-8 glasses/day to start
So now you've got the basic idea of what your body needs to survive. So where to plants fit in here?

Plants and Carbohydrates

Plants will help to provide your body with macronutrients it needs to function optimally. Plant-based foods including bananas, sweet potatoes, apples, pears and spinach, are quite high in carbs, more so than protein or fat. Since carbohydrates are the main source of energy for your cells it's important you get enough carbs into your diet. Experts agree that up to 65% of your caloric intake should come from carbohydrate sources, which is quite simple to do when choosing whole food options.

Plants and Protein

If you are eating animal foods like meat, eggs and dairy products, you will give your body complete proteins, meaning they give your body all the 20 essential amino acids in one shot. You can give your body all the protein it requires without using animal products, but you are going to have to combine various foods because none of these plant-based foods have complete proteins providing each of the 20 amino acids.

It may be a little bit more difficult, but it certainly doesn't take too long to get used to putting the puzzle pieces together. This just means you need to eat a variety of protein rich plant foods throughout the day to make sure you get your protein. An example might be eating some brown rice or pasta at lunch and having some chick peas at dinner. Perhaps you want to have some legumes for a snack and a handful of nuts after dinner. Diversity is key here and so long as you are eating a wide variety of colorful and protein rich plant-based foods daily you will keep on top of your bodily protein needs.

Quinoa is an exception to the rule. It is the only complete protein that is plant based.
Experts agree that up to 35% of your daily calories should come from protein.

Fiber and Plants

Fiber is one component of healthy eating you don't have to worry about lacking with plants. Plants are loaded with healthy fiber that helps to regulate your bodily systems

29

and naturally remove toxic buildup. Eliminating waste is only going to help your body function with more gusto.

There are two main types of fiber; soluble and insoluble Soluble fiber comes mainly from oats and fruits and helps to slow your digestive process down, making you feel fuller longer. This also allows for better nutrient absorption.

Insoluble fiber is abundant in natural veggies and grains and helps to increase the speed of digestion, helping to push waste out faster and keeping your internal systems functioning smoothly.

Nutritionists suggest about 15 grams of fiber for each thousand calories consumed is adequate.

Plants and Minerals

Plants offer all sorts of important minerals you need each day. Minerals are simply non-living substances that infiltrate into plants through the soil. Magnesium is plentiful in legumes and whole grains, necessary for nerve and muscle function. Phosphorus is found in various nuts and beans, helping to strengthen tissues and bones. Potassium is abundant in bananas, helping to regulate electrolytes and support cellular fluid function important in heart and muscle function and regulation.

Vitamins and Plants

Vitamins are living and made by plants. Vitamins are a must to maintain good health. Vitamin A is found in leafy green veggies, helping to keep your eyes healthy. Broccoli, strawberries and oranges are loaded with Vitamin C, strengthening your immune systems to start. Healthy whole grains are loaded with heart healthy B Vitamins, gather energy from the macronutrients to help your internal systems function effectively.

My Thoughts . . .
With knowledge and an open mind you can definitely get all the essential nutrients your body requires from a Whole Foods Plant Based Diet. In doing so you are choosing to fuel your body naturally without the interference harmful processing serves up. Energy levels will rise, fat will disappear, thinking will get crisper, chronic symptoms will lessen or disappear and disease will be avoided. Prevention is key to good health and choosing to stick with Mother Nature when fueling your body is going to push your health straight up to the top!

Sample Eating

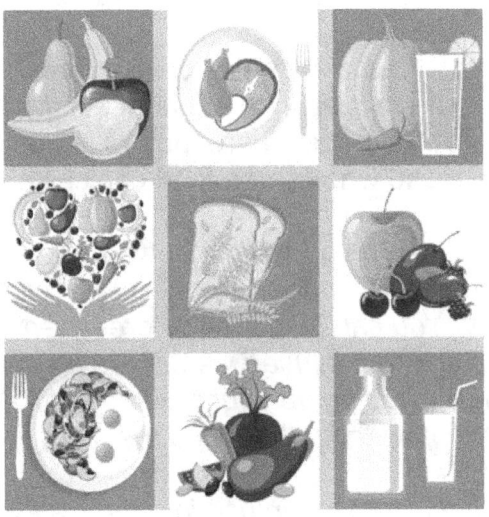

If you didn't know this already, your health and wellness, your life attitude, life decisions, energy levels, positivity and quality of life ARE dependent on how you fuel your body. The foods you choose to eat, in what quantity and when are all factors in how you are going to look, feel, act, think and perceive things.

Choosing natural energizing whole foods when you can is going to help you show your mind and body that you care about yourself. That you are looking to make the most of life and understand a strong body, void of disease, and a clear mind, sharp and effective, are MUSTS in the game of life. If you don't take care of your mental and physical, they aren't going to take care of you.

Avoiding convenient processed and packaged nutrient-poor foods is very important in healthy Whole Foods

Plant Based Diet eating. Plenty of fresh fruits and vegetables, whole grains, nuts, lean meats, fish, poultry, legumes and eggs are smart options, giving your body all the nutrients it requires to keep your body lean and strong and excited to stand the test of time.

Whole food choices and getting back with nature and pure goodness is a step in the right direction. Don't expect yourself to be perfect here, but it's important to do your best to make wholesome food choices always.

Drink Note - Ensure you carry a bottle of pure water around with you. It's important you get 6-8 glasses of water each day. You can also include green tea and herbal teas and natural fruit infused waters are also excellent. This just means slicing up your favorite fruits and putting them in a jug of water in the fridge the night before.

Overnight the flavors will infuse into the water and this makes a delicious all-natural beverage to make water a little more exciting. Stay away from caffeinated drinks, sodas and fruit juices that are loaded with sugars, additives and no nutrients.

Here are a few sample meals that will help you transition your mind and your actions towards healthier and wholesome.

Breakfast

It's the most important meal of the day. Your body has been on autopilot all night and is depleted of essential vitamins and minerals, vital nutrients it needs to function optimally. Eating a wholesome, healthy breakfast BEFORE you set your foot out the door, is an action that needs to be practice and practiced until it becomes habit. There's no room for excuses here.

Choice One

Instead of having a boxed cereal breakfast of package of quick ready oats, start your day with an omelet of free-range eggs, fresh herbs, spinach, tomato, onion, peppers and Parmesan cheese.

You'll need foods that are natural and wholesome, having been around back in the days when our ancestors were eating so healthy and natural. These foods provide just the right amount of healthy fats that aren't going to add fat to your frame, but rather help your body better absorb all the vitamins and minerals it requires to shine.

Choice Two

How about a dish of whole unpasteurized yogurt with loads of fresh berries and sprinkled with almonds? This provides the protein and good carbs your body needs to build lean muscle, increase your metabolism or rate in which you burn fat and starve off disease with those protective antioxidants from fresh berries. Of course, almonds also provide you with just enough fat to give you energy and help your thinking stay clear.

Lunch and Supper

What many people don't realize is that your body works best on a schedule. It likes to know when you will be eating for the most part so it can adjust what it needs to accomplish accordingly. Skipping meals and starving your body is all wrong. This is what screws up the smooth running of your internal systems, short-circuits your brain and causes negative interference that will give you loads of illness and disease, both mental and physical.

Intermittent eating mucks up your sleep schedule, triggers anxiety, turns off your natural fat burning hormones and makes you lazy and tired. Not eating will drop your blood sugar levels down dangerously low so that when you do eat, particularly if you are eating junk, your sugar levels will shoot straight to the top and this ping-pong action has been proven to trigger diabetes or at least increase your risk, not to mention more nasty mood swings and complete rewiring of your system and not for the better. Do yourself a favor. Listen to your body and eat when it needs it. Next, make sure you give it whole foods so it can get the job done, which of course is helping you to look fantastic, feel great and have ample energy on tap!

Making sure you get fuel your body here with lean protein, vegetables and good fat is going to set your body up to smile.

Choice One

For lunch have a spinach salad with grilled free-range chicken, tomato, cucumber, onion, sesame seeds, sunflowers seeds and a drizzle of coconut oil-based dressing.

For dinner grill a salmon steak with a drizzle of olive oil and fresh herbs, grilled sweet potato, sliced avocado and steamed broccoli, kale, carrots, peas, beans and water chestnuts. Natural organic whole grain bread goes nicely with this.

Choice Two

For lunch try placing a cup of quinoa into a Romaine leaf for a wrap. You can add tomato and cucumber. A cup of unpasteurized whole yogurt with sliced banana, mango and crushed almonds tops it off perfectly.

For dinner grill a chicken breast drizzled in soybean oil and fresh herbs. Steam parsnip, broccoli, spinach, peppers and eggplant and lentils for a nutritious side loaded with protein for calorie burning, carbs for long-lasting energy and essential vitamins and minerals to support your internal systems and their function.

Snacking

Unfortunately, we're conditioned to view snacking as devilish, sneaky and unhealthy. Snacking is often choosing processed sweet foods that are high in bad fat, sugars and calories and have very little nutritional gain. This includes chips, cookies, muffins, French fries, chocolate bars and other sweets.

These food choices blast us with short-lived energy because of the massive dose of sugar and leave us hungrier lickety-split!

Here are a few excellent whole food options to wrap your head around that will give you the energy you are searching for and the staying power that makes it "sweet"

* Handful of nuts and dried fruit (careful not to overdose because a serving is 2-3 tbsp), gives you the protein and good fats your mind and body needs

* Hardboiled eggs and raw veggies, gives you protein, iron and the fiber your body needs to naturally get rid of toxic buildup

* Celery and all-natural peanut butter, fiber, protein for energy and good fats in perfect combination

* Sliced avocado on fresh fruit and veggies, healthy fats, protein, carbohydrates, vitamins and minerals to help build your body and mind strong

* Fruit salad with plenty of berries, talk about a protective punch

* Handful of raisins and organic kale chips, vitamins and minerals to energize

* Sliced sweet potato crisps, slice sweet potatoes, sprinkle with herbs and back until crisp

* All-natural beef jerky will give your body a quick dose of protein without the fuss

* All-natural fruit juice smoothie make with almond milk, dates, and fruits of your choice, fat metabolizing energy with staying power

My Thoughts . . .
Whole food eating doesn't have to be difficult. In fact it's our high-tech fast food eating that is causing all the ruckus. Taking the time to "tell" yourself all the positives of eating whole foods is the first step in the transformation process. Set yourself up for success by trying something you can see yourself enjoying. In other words consider your preferences and tolerances in all food choices and open your mind to change. One step at a time and allow yourself to take a step backwards here and there, you're only human.

You never know unless you try and by using these meal and snack ideas as a guide you will find what words for your body mentally and physical. The approach has to be married or it just won't work.

Disease Prevention and Whole Food Connection

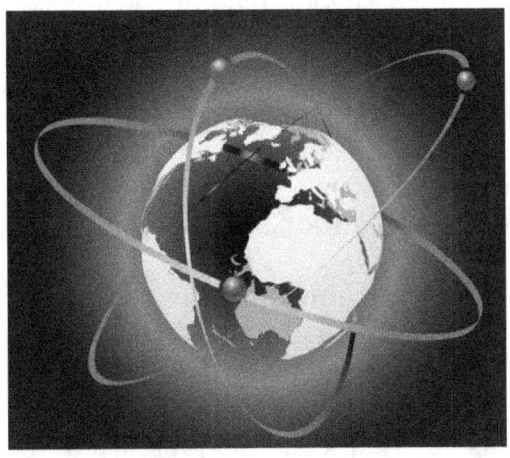

So why is it important you eat healthier by choosing natural whole foods?

* Prevents bone and muscle loss and vitamin deficiency that will result in serious disease and chronic conditions

* Disease prevention including cancer, stroke, cardiovascular disease, diabetes and osteoporosis to start

* Naturally lowers high blood pressure and the risk for celiac disease and diabetes

In order to maintain good health you have to give your body all the macro and micronutrients it requires. If you survive on processed fast foods there is ZERO chance you will stay healthy. It's only a matter of time before you trigger illness and disease that will eventually take your life.

Adequate amounts of protein, carbohydrates, fats, vitamins, minerals and water are critical in keeping your organs and internal systems functioning optimally. This includes the health of your mind because if your physical isn't healthy your mind is truly mucked up.

Take note vitamins and minerals come from all-natural substances necessary for your good health. They are need for physical function, thinking and the metabolic process that breaks down flabby fat.

Disease Prevention and Control

PREVENTION is everything in life. Just think about it from a practical perspective. If you happen to be goofing off and break your leg, you can get it "fixed," but it's still never going to be the same.

Regardless of how skilled the surgeon that set your bone or how fabulous your physical therapist was, your leg will never be as healthy or strong as it was. A break is a break and this means your leg is weaker than it was before you broke it up, even after it's completely healed. As years go on your break may come back and bug you because of chronic aches and pains or perhaps the break was bad enough that it threw off your bodily alignment, causing you to favor one side. Over time, this might very well develop into a limp and the side effects snowball from there.

Well, the same thing applies with disease. If you can prevent disease with healthy and energizing whole food choices why wouldn't you? Do you want to have to control symptoms after the fact for the rest of your life?

Wouldn't you rather make the changes now so you don't ever have to experience heart disease, stroke, diabetes or any other sickness?

Experts agree that whole food eating is the best choice you can make for your body. It's all about perspective here, give and take. You don't have to be perfect and make a whole food choice EVERY time. The idea is to re-teach yourself how to eat and eventually you are going to WANT to eat an apple instead of a bag of potato chips. A grilled chicken with steamed asparagus and cauliflower is going to make your mouth water instead of a greasy burger and fries.

It's all about DECIDING to make a change for the better and committing to it. It's setting yourself up for success, practicing and giving it time to sink in. You CAN do it if you want.

Would you agree that obesity is the root of most evil and preventable disease? I set you up for success here, so if you didn't get that one right it's all your fault. Scientists agree that losing weight, even just a few pounds, will greatly reduce your risk of developing all sorts of serious disease. By simply choosing to eat less high-energy-dense foods and more low-energy-dense foods you are increases the ability for your body to burn fat and lose weight.

High-energy-dense foods are processed foods, fried foods, sweets, full fat salad dressings and other devilish delights, often loaded with saturated fats and high cho-lesterol that doesn't do your body good. Lower calorie foods with ample nutrients is what you want to load your body with and this is what you'll find with low-energy-dense food options.

Low-energy-dense foods are healthy choices including fresh vegetables and fruit.

The "Dietary Guide for Americans" suggests a healthy whole food diet should consist of:

* Focusing on fresh fruits and vegetables, whole grains and milk products

* Adequate amounts of lean meats, fish, skinless chicken and turkey, nuts, eggs and beans

* Include sparing amounts of healthy unsaturated fats, be low in cholesterol, avoid saturated and Trans fat as much as possible, void of added sugars and little sodium

Disease prevention BEGINS with fueling your body right, which also helps naturally remove toxic buildup from your system that triggers disease and illness. Processed and packaged foods have chemicals and preservatives your body doesn't know how to flush from your system. Over time this builds up and interferes with good health.

Choosing whole foods and drinking plenty of water is a natural way to give your body the nutrients it needs to fight disease and the liquid and fiber necessary to purge toxins.

Fabulous Disease Fighting Whole Foods

Fatty Fish
In fatty fish like tuna and salmon, you'll find omega 3 fatty acids which help naturally lower blood fats, preventing blood clots from developing that are symptoms of heart disease. Studies show that having fatty fish twice a week lowers your risk of heart disease tremendously.

Sweet Potato

Sweet potatoes are loaded with protective antioxidants, beta-carotene, E and C vitamins, folate, iron, copper, calcium and potassium. There are nice quantities of fiber that encourage a healthy digestive system and the protective antioxidants help prevent cancer and cardiovascular disease.

Various Nuts

Nuts are tasty treats that give your body the healthy fat it requires to function optimally. This fat helps lower cholesterol natural which is a trigger for a variety of serious disease. Nuts also have plenty of:
* fiber
* protein
* E and A vitamins
* selenium
Nuts are a great energy dense snack to hold you over, but you do have to be careful because they are very high in calories and good fat. A handful is lots for a serving.

Eggs

Eggs are one of the best sources of protein and have essential vitamins and minerals necessary for good eye health. The choline in eggs is an essential nutrient, particularly for pregnant women. Eggs are easy to eat and fit into any meal and as with any food, if you eat them sensibly, they're only going to do your body good.
An egg a day will help keep the doctor away.

Spinach, Romaine and Others Greens

Your bests whole foods to deter disease are a wide array of leafy green veggies. Packed full of minerals, essential vitamins, vitamin C, magnesium, phytochemicals, antioxidants, iron, folate, fiber and so much more, it makes sense to load your plate up.

Experts suggest eating a diet with magnesium is going to help lower your risk of developing diabetes. Spinach has lots of magnesium.

My Thoughts . . .
In general fruits and vegetables are the "powerhouses" of disease fighting and prevention nutrients, some of which are an array of minerals, vitamins, fiber, antioxidants and phytochemicals. The jury is out on this and ensuring you get at least 5-6 servings a day is going to help lower your risk of cancer and numerous other diseases. Choosing to bypass processed foods and throwing refined eating out the window and replace it with whole food plant based eating is only going to give your body and mind a fighting chance. The choice as always is yours.

Exercising and Whole Foods

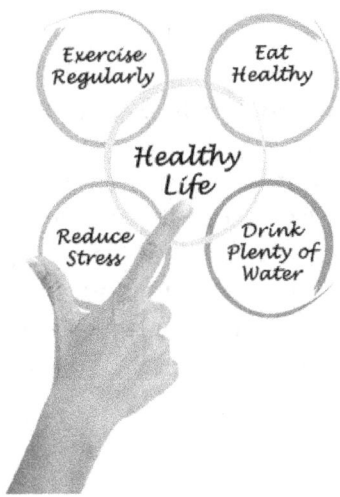

Do you want to exercise with your tank half empty or full to the brim? Would you prefer clean pure energy that lasts or intermittent bursts of highs and lows when exercising?

If you eat foods that are loaded with harmful fats, sugars and calories, you are not going to exercise effectively and efficiently to burn off pesky fat stores. Processed fast foods, pastries and sweets give your body FAST energy that goes as quickly as it came. This energy is not useful for the body. It's the wrong fuel for your body to convert into energy to maximize fat burn and energy gain.

If you want to increase your metabolism by exercising AND burn off the fat that is stored, you need to give your body adequate amounts of good fat, lean protein and complex carbohydrates. These macronutrients don't come from nutrition-less fast foods that are fried and come in boxes. You need to build lean muscle to burn fat, and if you are building muscle with exercising you need protein.

Before and After Exercising

You should have a snack with protein and complex carbohydrates to help give your system the nutrition it needs to build lean muscle and zap fat. Of course always drinking plenty of water to ensure the essential macronutrients, vitamins and minerals get dispersed throughout your body for maximized energy and results. This is also important after you have finished exercising because you need to replenish your vitamin stores.

Sample Snacks

* Apples dipped in all-natural peanut butter are a perfect protein and carbohydrate rich snack to give your body the energy it requires to exercise. A whole grain bagel with peanut butter also works nicely about an hour before training and immediately after.

* All-natural energy bars that are 70% carbohydrates and 30% protein are also an excellent choice. Just be sure you don't choose one with excess sugar added.

* Fresh veggies and hummus is the perfect energizer when exercising. The vegetables give you the fiber, carbohydrates and antioxidant protection, while protein storage is taken care of with the hummus. About half a cup of hummus with about a cup of veggies should do the trick.

* If you're really in a pinch a handful of nuts should do the trick. This will give your body fast access to easily absorbed protein, omega-3s, vitamin E, selenium and your carb needs are satisfied too.

* Tossing a grilled chicken breast in a Romaine lettuce leaf with about a 1/4 cup of quinoa is tasty, and it gives your body and mind the energy to perform. This can be eaten cold and works really well when trying to eat up the leftovers from dinner.

* Peanut butter and banana on whole grain bread or crackers is another snack that packs a punch. You should use a 1-2 tbsp of peanut butter, half a banana and one piece of whole grain bread or 6-8 crackers.

Your body is a machine that is dependent on a wide array of nutrients so function optimally. If you deprive your body of what it needs to formulate new cells, repair damaged ones, work all your internal organs and ensure all the receptors in your body are working well, you will run into trouble in time. Usually your body grabs your attention with aches, pains and disease. We usually just ignore it and let it manifest into something permanent that takes away from our quality of life.
The choice is yours.

How much should you exercise?

Of course this is a subjective question, but most experts agree that people should do some sort of exercising every day. What's more important though, is that you set yourself up for success, because something is better than nothing. Always consider your preferences and tolerances before you get started.

30-45 minutes of moderate to intense cardiovascular activity 3-5 days a week is a great place to start. Add to that 2-3 days of strength training or weight lifting for 15 minutes each time and you should be good to go. Honestly, it really doesn't take a whole lot of time to keep your body in shape physically if you commit to exercising smart. You do not have to be a gym rat to get physically healthy.

Find the activities you enjoy!

If you can't stand going to the gym then maybe you want to ride your bike and lift some light weights at home? Perhaps swimming is something you love? If you love classes, a boot camp training session three times a week for an hour each time is all you need to get fit! These classes maximize the energy you burn and are probably one of the "best" forms of exercise out there. Boot camp session use an interval training method that keeps your mind and body guessing, which means you are never going to get bored and both physically and mentally you will always be challenged.

Boot camp sessions challenge you each class to work harder than you did the class before. You are in competition with yourself amongst a group of varying skill levels. These classes alternate periods of high intensity and low intensity cardiovascular, muscular and stretching and toning exercising to keep your heart rate up and fat burning off.

It's the diversity of these sessions that make them so effective. Exercises are always changing along with intensity, weight, reps, duration, pace and pattern. You might as well make the most of your exercise time right?

You run on other people's energy because each is always pushing to do their very best and fat loss, lean muscle gain and a beautiful toned and healthy body is the result. It's pretty tough not to get caught up in the positive adrenaline when it's all around you!

The best part of all is that you work at your level always, and it's the instructors that continuously push all the right buttons for you to do better each time. This means more fat loss, improved self-confidence and a leaner, stronger, happier you.

Eating a well- balanced diet with the right amount of protein, carbohydrates, good fat, vitamins and minerals and drinking plenty of pure water, is going to set your body up to burn fat, build lean muscle and feel like a million bucks; mind, body and soul.

My Thinking . . .
Without a healthy "physical" body you are sunk. Every single thing you do is dependent on being physically able, even if you want to smile you've got to use your facial muscles and mind to do so. This takes energy and means your body needs to use up some of the energy you have given it. This energy needs to be replenished, and when you are exercising you really need to pay attention because you are using more energy in the form of protein, carbohydrates and fats, to give your body the ability to work hard for you. If the energy isn't there and you are still trying to exercise, stress is caused and this will negatively affect you.

Did you know that if you are training and don't get enough protein from your body to use for muscle formation and bodily function, your body will actually break down the muscle you have already worked hard to build

and use it as energy. This is choice number one regard-
less of how much fat you are carrying around.

If you want to burn off fat, you have to eat and make sure
your body has enough lean protein and complex carbo-
hydrates to give your body the ability to burn fat off.
When fat storages are topped off, all you have to worry
about is actually implementing the physical exercise.
Your body will take care of the rest.

Your body is uniquely complex and it's in your best inter-
ests to do your best to make sure your body has the
optimal energy that it requires to exercise. Whole food
eating in the "right" combinations is going to set you up to
build your body lean while keeping your energy levels
happy and high.
Once again the choice is yours.

Whole Foods and the Mental Benefits

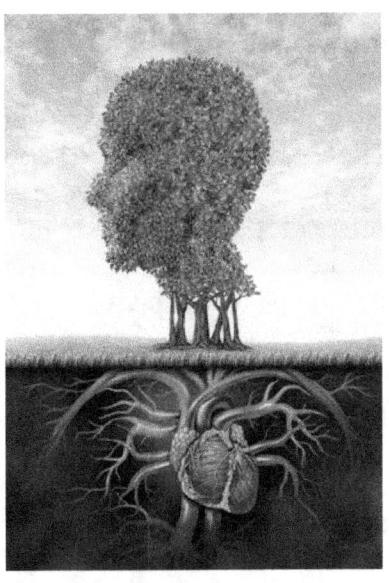

When it comes to getting healthy we often focus solely on the physical. Many assume that if you are in shape physically you are healthy and often this just isn't the case. Your good health is dependent on both physical and mental. You can't really have one without the other.

Your mind is a powerful thing. It controls your reality, how you perceive life in general and whether or not you are going to commit to getting healthy for life and feeling great about it, or quit. It's the mind that dictates your actions and making sure your "mental" or thinking is optimal will only help you reach your goals faster and more effectively.

What good is it to have a six pack and be physically strong if you are always depressed and unhappy with you? Is it so much so that you stay inside your house most days anyway? Making healthy whole food choices is only going to help your mind and body function as one, which is necessary for optimal health.

Fact: It goes without saying that what you eat directly affects your mood tremendously.

Your diet also affects how you act and your internal brain function. If you aren't eating well, your energy levels are likely see-sawing, on top of the world one minute and de-pressingly devastated the next. If you are choosing to eat junk food meals you will rarely be satisfied for long.

Loads of sugars and unhealthy fats into your system in large doses is going to leave you hungry and unsatisfied all the time and because of the preservative and harmful chemical interference you are going to have all sorts of troubles, from sleep issues, to skin breakouts, extreme fatigue and emotional chaos. Food is a very important player in how your see yourself, your life attitude, pas-sions and ability to think clearly and with effectiveness. Understanding which foods are best not only for your physical well- being, but also your mental is top priority. You are worth it!

Nutritional factors influencing your emotional well-being

* Protein intake
* Carbohydrate intake
* Fat intake
* Vitamins, minerals and alcohol intake
* Total amount of energy you take in
* Genetic composition and medical status

Even if you are missing a single vitamin your brain function may be negatively affected.

Examples of how your eating habits affect mood

* Highs and lows of blood sugar levels

* Not getting enough vitamins and minerals or fatty acids can disturb your thinking

* The foods you eat directly affect your brain function

* Specific nutrients missing can directly affect your ability to digest food and convert it into energy

* Breathing in unclear air can interfere with your brain and physical function

* Preservatives, bad fats and other harmful chemicals added to food can affect your brain, manifest over time and create disease

One deadly habit that affects far too many people is depending on fast food eating to fuel the body. Fat foods are anything, but good for your body or thinking, loaded with saturated fats, calories, salt and harmful chemicals that will build up over time in your internal organs and start causing issue. Lipids build up in the blood over time increasing sugar in your blood tax your pancreas and liver, increasing your risk of developing diabetes.

This sort of unhealthy eating stressing your body and mind and slowly, but surely you will poison yourself from the inside out. Choosing not to give your body and mind the clean whole foods it craves will come with a price. Is this a price you want to have to pay? Is your good health really worth a few fries and greasy burgers?

Mental clarity and eating

Iron

If you don't give your body enough iron, you will feel extremely fatigued and often ill. Not having enough iron in your bloodstream will leave you without energy and this causes your body stress. By choosing to eat whole and healthy dark leafy green veggies, whole grains, beans and eggs, you will provide your body with the nutrient it needs to get healthy mentally and physically.

Folic Acid

If you aren't getting enough folic acid you may be moody, tired, not hungry, and have trouble sleeping. Women that are pregnant need to make certain they have ample folic acid because it's critical in normal baby formation. Eating whole foods including beans, peas, spinach. squash and raisins is a good way to boost your stores. Doctors recommend pregnant women take a multivitamin with folic acid just to be sure.

Omega 3s

Omega 3 fatty acids are important for decreasing cholesterol, sharpening the mind and preventing cardiovascular disease. Fatty fish like salmon, tuna and cod are great sources and experts recommend you eat fish twice a week. Studies show that increasing your omega 3s will help improve brain function.

Zinc

Zinc is found in liver, eggs, seafood, numerous veggies and red meat. If you don't get enough zinc irreversible neurological damage may occur. Not getting enough may lead to the jitters, grumpiness and extreme tiredness.

B Vitamins

Too much stress and drinking excessive amounts of alcohol will interfere with B vitamin storage and use. Not enough of these vitamins will make you really tired, grumpy, moody, and you may not be able to sleep. Eating plenty of healthy whole grains, nuts, legumes, seeds and organ meats will give your body adequate amounts. Milk, eggs and animals meats are also excellent sources.

Selenium
In order for hormones to be synthesized selenium is required. This also helps protect membranes from getting damaged. By eating plenty of seeds, nuts, eggs, grains and seafood, you should be able to give your body adequate amounts of selenium for optimal mental and physical function

My Thoughts . . .
As you can see your mental health is just as important as the physical in the big picture. Both are intricately connected and don't function well separately. Eating whole foods is going to give your mind and body the "right" amount of optimal nutrients to give you the energy you need to support your body and mind and function at the top of your game. This means that you will have the ability to deter disease, feel and look like a million bucks and maybe even walk around with a skip in your step.

Final Thoughts

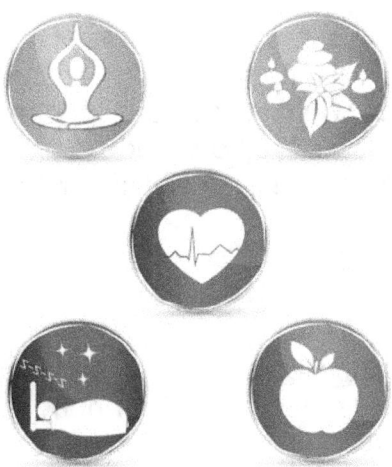

Eating whole foods is pretty tough to argue because this is what nature intended, natural, virgin, nutrient rich foods that are easily absorbed by the body, providing the perfect energy required to function optimally mentally and physically. Progress and technology really has messed this perfect concept up and caused harmful and often deadly interference.

As a fast paced society, we have learned to make unhealthy processed food eating habit. Habits are hard to break especially when our mind and senses tell us this one tastes really good.

We teach our body and mind to crave sweet and nutrition-less convenience foods and allow our emotions and life stresses to dictate what we eat and how much. We use things such as heartache and depression to deem valid the need for a chocolate bar or tub of ice cream instead of teach ourselves to go for a fun or grab an apple. Not an apple fritter, slice of apple pie or an apple muffin, but a real life wholesome and natural apple, picked right of the tree is preferable.

We get used to this destructive cycle of habitual remorse, and just accept it as "normal." As a lazy society unaccustomed to change we allow overeating, obesity and all sorts of other nasty conditions and circumstances to manifest. It looks to me like we just don't care. You are in charge of you right?

Action Steps . . .
First . . .
You need to acknowledge and accept change needs to happen if you are going to get your body healthier mentally and physically.

Second . . .
You need to understand that whole food eating is the best route to provide your body with the essential macronutrients and micronutrients it needs to give you energy, deter disease, burn fat, build lean muscle and leave you feeling healthy and happy mentally, physically, spiritually and emotionally.

Third . . .
You need to commit to gaining knowledge about whole foods in general, which ones work best with your preferences and tolerances , making sure you keep an open mind to try new things and always keep yourself moving forward.

Fourth . . .
Make the changes necessary for you start reaping the rewards. Set yourself up for success by implementing changes slowly so they can be managed. Too much too

soon will result in you falling backwards into your un-healthy, but comfortable ways of days past.

Perhaps you want to start with skipping your afternoon vending machine snack, and opting for a handful of nuts or a couple pieces of fresh fruit? Instead of having white toast with butter for breakfast, have whole grain toast with peanut butter. It's so important you make managea-ble changes that make sense to you and that you WANT to truly commit to for life.

This is not a fad diet that comes and goes. This is all about making the changes that stick and that part is all up to you. Go big or go home doesn't play in this park.

Fifth . . .
Actually set up your meal plans at least the day before. So you know what foods you need to buy and you don't waste time trying to figure it out when you're hungry. That can get you into big trouble.

Sixth . . .
Make sure you experiment and figure out what sort of physical exercise fits best for your daily activity. Start off slow and work your way forward, always checking with your healthcare provider first just to be safe. It's so im-portant you enjoy the exercise you choose if you want to implement and solidify it long term, remembering your best option is to use both cardiovascular and muscle building exercises and always change it up.

Seventh . . .
This one is the most important of all. Commit to NEVER quitting. The only way you can fail with the Whole Foods Plant Based Diet is to actually throw in the towel. There will be setbacks and it's important you accept this. Most importantly you need to accept them, let them go and

move forward. You're human and "mistakes" will happen. Onward all eyes forward is your first option.

Take the knowledge you've gained and apply it to your personal tastes, preferences, tolerances and life beliefs. Healthy Whole foods are what Mother Nature tells us to eat. It's really tough to re-program our thinking from what we know and have been taught. Technology, convenience, more money, less sleep, more "toys," faster cars have slowly, but surely made their way into our lives and pushed away the basics, things like eating healthy whole foods, entertaining ourselves with good old endorphin releasing exercise. When stressed, go for a run instead of drowning our sorrows in a tub of double chocolate sugar loaded ice cream while watching our favorite television program.

The price we pay for all these convenient luxuries in life is our health. That's ironic seeing as your health is the most important asset you own. It's time to make a natural and wholesome change for the better one step at a time, don't you think?

We have the choice to look for the positive or the negative in life. You can choose to lift someone up or to stomp on them. Writing is my passion and I work hard at it, with the goal of helping make people better. If you gain a new piece of knowledge, read something that makes you think, or perhaps even smile a few times, then I am happy and content!

Life's just too short not to tune into optimism. If your glass is half full, then I invite you to read my writing, and if you have a minute to spare when you're through, **I would appreciate your review.** This will help me better myself and my writing. I thank you in advance and appreciate you.